I0464624

1

SLAYING THE HIDDEN DRAGON

Living or dying with HEPATITIS C / HCV

BETTER ME THAN YOU

This book is dedicated to my Sister, My wife, my family and the millions of people affected by **THE SILENT DRAGON**. Better known as **HEPATITIS C.** I am just one of millions of BABY BOOMERS out there who has been infected with the debilitating disease / virus known as Hepatitis C or HCV. My very survival to this day is accredited to **God**, my Wife at the time, my family and the professional health care staff at the world famous MAYO CLINIC. Without the support of these remarkable individuals, I would not be here today.

By reading this book you will understand how important it is to safeguard yourself and survive in the event that you have been introduced to the **Hidden Dragon**. There are not many people out there who could survive what I HAVE BEEN THROUGH. If I can help anyone in any way by publishing this story, and prevent them from the perils I have been through, I will consider this effort a success.

MYTHS: There is only one way to contact HCV. This is by direct blood to blood exposure. The virus cannot be spread by kissing, casual contact, drinking from the same glass, swimming in the same water, wearing the same clothes, or through food preparation or sharing.

Transmission: The hepatitis C virus is a blood borne virus. It is most commonly transmitted through:

1. Injecting drug use through the sharing of injection equipment.

2. In health care settings due to the reuse or inadequate sterilization of medical equipment, especially syringes and needles.

3. In many cases before 1993, HCV was transmitted via the transfusion of unscreened blood and blood products.

4. Hepatitis C is not spread through breast milk, food or water or by casual contact such as hugging, kissing and sharing food or drinks with an infected person.

5. The **Hidden Dragon** can be transmitted through sex. However, it is extremely rare and there has to be direct blood to blood contact.

I have been married and have never spread the virus. Infection through sex is very rare. In my case, I was infected by a blood transfusion in 1972 when I was sixteen years old. The virus remained in my system for 37 years with no symptoms or signs of ill health.

If you received a blood transfusion before 1993 it would be in your best interest to get checked. It is possible to lead a healthy and productive life after diagnosis by leading a healthy lifestyle. As long as cirrhosis or kidney failure has not set in.

All medical terms and procedures are explained here to the best of my ability. I am in no way a Doctor or a Medical Professional. However, I am a prime example of survival. We as Human Beings are complex life forms that have been graced with the basic ability to reason, research, make our own decisions and use common sense. When we lose these abilities we need help. Fortunately for me, the recipe for survival came together.

CHAPTER ONE :

THE FIRST SIGNS

The year is 2009. I am married, living in a new house, I am a professional in the field of Recreational Water. Swimming Pools, Fountains, Spas, anything with water in it. I can fix, maintain or trouble shoot just about anything related to recreational water. I have been a professional Bartender, Half ass Musician "Drummer", Food and Beverage Professional and free lance Photographer for my entire life. While unloading my tool box off of my trailer I slipped and miss stepped, blowing out my knee from an old sports injury thirty years prior. Man, let me tell you how bad it hurt. I was hobbling around thinking it was going to heal. Being a big, strong guy I was not too concerned. However, as days passed it got worse and I began to wonder.

My Wife suggested I go in for a physical. I had not seen a doctor in quite some time and she is a very convincing, beautiful gal. Guys do not go to the doctor unless something hurts. Her suggestion saved my life. I bought a knee brace and continued to work. It was uncomfortable but nothing was going to keep me away from the work that I was so passionate about. A few days later the doctor called with results. He told me that my liver enzymes were elevated, and that my ACL was severed. Your ACL is a tendon. The **Anterior Cruciate Ligament** runs diagonally in the middle of the knee. It prevents the tibia from sliding out in front of the femur, as well as provides rotational stability to the knee.

I realized that my knee was in a lot worse shape than I thought. I was then referred to a **gastrointestinologist,** who is a specialist in studying the ailment and problems mainly related to intestines.

It was this Doctor who diagnosed me with HCV. At this point I was still A-symptomatic and felt great. However, my liver enzymes were high and my blood count was off. The white blood cells that fight off infection and disease were low, and I needed surgery on my knee. Not only does the **Hidden Dragon** affect your white blood cell count, it also affects your platelet Count.

Thrombocytopenia is the medical term for a low blood platelet count. **Platelets** (thrombocytes) are colorless blood cells that play an important role in blood clotting. Platelets stop blood loss by clumping and forming plugs in blood vessel holes.

Thrombocytopenia often occurs as a result of a separate disorder, such as leukemia or an immune system problem such as HCV, or as a medication side effect.

Thrombocytopenia may be mild and cause few signs or symptoms. In rare cases, the number of platelets may be so low that dangerous internal bleeding can occur. Thrombocytopenia usually improves when the underlying cause is treated. Sometimes medications, surgery or a blood transfusion can help treat chronic thrombocytopenia.

At this point I went in to an orthopedic surgeon concerning my knee. It was August 2009 when the doctor performed my ACL replacement surgery. After extensive blood tests, x-rays and CT scans, the Doctor approved my operation. I healed fast and was back to work within nine weeks. For the next two years I felt fabulous and continued to work full time. When the seasonal swimming pool work slumped off for the Resort I was working for I did my own thing, making a living independently as a certified swimming pool repair tech.

Then in March, 2011 I was offered a job as General Mgr. of a local Steakhouse / Saloon.

I figured I had been doing the heavy construction and maintenance thing long enough. Time to slow down a little and go back to my food and beverage roots.

Man, I tell you. Life was good. Once again I was doing a job that I totally enjoyed and was passionate about. Then in June 2011 it happened. I woke up one morning and my stomach was swollen up. I literally looked like I had swallowed a basketball. My ankles and lower legs were also swollen. I was constipated and weak. I could not stay up on my feet for longer than 45 minutes at a time. I went from acute diarrhea to constipation on a daily basis and my skin was blotched with red spots covering my whole body. So back to the Doctor it was. This was the beginning of the symptoms. I had been feeling so good, and was so happy.

Come to find out, the swelling in my stomach was diagnosed as **ascites**. When fluid builds up inside the abdomen, it is known as ascites.

Ascites usually occurs when the liver stops working properly. Fluid fills the space between the lining of the abdomen and the organs. Ascites is most often caused by liver scarring. This increases pressure inside the liver's blood vessels. The increased pressure can force fluid into the abdominal cavity, causing ascites. Liver damage is the biggest risk factor for ascites. Some causes of liver damage include cirrhosis, hepatitis b or c or a history of heavy alcohol abuse. People with ascites only have a five-year survival rate of 30 to 40 percent. If you experience ascites symptoms, talk to your doctor as soon as possible. Diagnosing ascites takes multiple steps. Your doctor will first check for swelling in your abdomen. Then he will probably use imaging to look for fluid.

Abdominal imaging might include an ultrasound, CT scan, or MRI. Blood tests, laparoscopy, and angiography can also be used to diagnose ascites.

The swelling of my ankles and lower legs was diagnosed as **peripheral adema**. Leg swelling caused by the retention of fluid in leg tissues is known as peripheral edema. It can be caused by a problem with the circulatory system, the lymphatic system or the kidneys. You may also experience swelling due to fluid buildup after sitting or standing for a long time. Factors related to fluid buildup include: Acute kidney failure / Cardiomyopathy (disease of heart tissue) / Chronic kidney disease / Cirrhosis / Nephrotic syndrome (damage to small filtering blood vessels in the kidneys), as well as several other disorders.

In my case, the **Hidden Dragon** had taken its toll. **Cirrhosis** had set in. I was experiencing end stage liver failure.

My doctor prescribed some specialty medications for me to try and help with these problems.

Spironolactone is a potassium-sparing diuretic (water pill) that prevents your body from absorbing too much salt and keeps your potassium levels from getting too low. **Spironolactone** is used to diagnose or treat a condition in which you have too much aldosterone in your body. **Aldosterone** is a hormone produced by your adrenal glands to help regulate the salt and water balance in your body. **Spironolactone** also treats fluid retention (edema) in people with congestive heart failure, cirrhosis of the liver, or a kidney disorder called nephrotic syndrome. This medication is also used to treat or prevent hypokalemia (low potassium levels in the blood).

Furosemide is a loop diuretic (water pill) that prevents your body from absorbing too much salt, allowing the salt to instead be passed in your urine.

Furosemide is also a drug that treats fluid retention. In my case I was prescribed both medications.

The swelling went down and I started feeling ok. Although tired and having problems with constipation, I was surviving.

Male Gynecomastia is no fun at all. In my case my breasts enlarged during treatment. It is uncomfortable and painful. **Gynecomastia** is a common clinical condition consisting of a benign proliferation of male breast glandular tissue. The symptom is pain and swelling of the breast. Gynecomastia itself is not a disease but, rather, a symptom of an underlying imbalance in hormonal physiology—specifically, an increase in estrogen action relative to androgen action at the breast tissue level.

Spironolactone is a potassium-holding diuretic used to treat ascites due to liver cirrhosis, and Gynecomastia is a well-known side effect of the medication.

If you get lucky the swelling will recede after treatment. However, in some cases the symptoms remain for life. **I got lucky**

BETTER ME THAN YOU

After a couple of months, in August 2011 my constipation was beginning to really bother me. Sometimes it would be 3 to 4 days without a bowel movement. Very painful and irritating indeed. The next medication prescribed was a specialty laxative called lactulose. **Lactulose** is a synthetic, non-digestible sugar used in the treatment of chronic constipation and **hepatic encephalopathy**. **Lactulose** is a thick syrup and has a horrid taste, and must be taken three times a day.

Lactulose takes two to three days to get in to your system. Your stomach cramps up and when it finally starts to work, look out. You better be close to a toilet.

A liver damaged by The **Silent Dragon / HCV** has trouble removing toxins from your body — normally one of the liver's key tasks.

The buildup of toxins can damage your brain, leading to changes in your mental state, behavior and personality (**hepatic encephalopathy**). Signs and symptoms of hepatic encephalopathy include forgetfulness, confusion and mood changes, and in the most severe cases, **coma**.

Within six months I was pretty much bed ridden. Leaving the house only for short trips to the store or for doctors appointments. Cramping in the legs and calves is almost too painful to handle. Sleep is almost impossible because of nocturnal pruritus.

Pruritus, or itch, is defined as an unpleasant sensation that provokes the desire to scratch.

Certain systemic diseases have long been known to cause pruritus that ranges in intensity from a mild annoyance to an intractable, disabling condition. Nocturnal pruritus only starts to itch when the body slows down and you try to go to sleep.

Pruritus is very annoying, and if you scratch it only gets worse. Then, with the compromised immune system, welts, scabs and open soars appear. The only relief is a sleeping agent. However, with the liver problems you cannot take any sleep aids or pain meds. Therefore sleep is never more than an hour or two at a time, at the most.

My Wife scheduled an appointment for me at the Mayo Clinic in Phoenix / Scottsdale Arizona. My initial appointment lasted ten days. The professional staff and technicians at Mayo Clinic are the best in the world.

The tests that were done and the information they provided was a little frightening but very informative. The Doctor prescribed me some special medications to try and kill the virus.

These drugs were a combination of injectables and oral medications.

Until a few years ago, there were only two drugs approved by the FDA for treating HCV. These drugs are:

- **Pegylated interferon**: Interferon is similar to a protein your body makes to fight off infection. Pegylated interferon or PEGASYS is a long acting form of interferon. It can be used alone, but is almost always used with Ribavirin.

- **Ribavirin**: This is used only in combination with interferon. It can never be used alone to treat Hepatitis C.

Combination therapy with pegylated interferon and ribavirin – often referred to as PEG/riba therapy – increases the chances of getting rid of the virus from your body.

In May 2011, the FDA approved two new medications that are part of a drug group called **protease inhibitors**.

These drugs are:

- **Boceprevir** (brand name **Victrelis**)
- **Telaprevir** (brand name **Incivek**)

These last two drugs show promise. They are orally administered. However, if your kidneys are not functioning at 40% or more these two drugs run a high risk of causing chronic kidney failure. The PEG/riba therapy was working ok. Injections had to be done on a daily basis along with the oral supplement. My **MELD** score was going down.

The **Model for End-Stage Liver Disease**, or **MELD** is a scoring system for assessing the severity of chronic liver disease. MELD was originally developed at the Mayo Clinic by Dr. Patrick Kamath, and at that point was called the "Mayo End-stage Liver Disease" score.

MELD uses the patient's values for serum bilirubin, serum creatinine, and the international normalized ratio for prothrombine time (INR) to predict survival.

Bilirubin (formerly referred to as **haematoidin**) is a yellow breakdown product of the human body, a principal component of red blood cells. Bilirubin is excreted in bile and urine, and elevated levels may indicate certain diseases. It is responsible for the yellow color of bruises, the background straw-yellow color of urine, the brown color of feces and the yellow discoloration in jaundice.

A **creatinine test** reveals important information about your kidneys.

Creatinine is a chemical waste product that is produced by your muscle metabolism and to a smaller extent by eating meat. Healthy kidneys filter creatinine and other waste products from your blood. The filtered waste products leave your body in your urine. If your kidneys aren't functioning properly, an increased level of **creatinine** may accumulate in your blood. A **serum creatinine** test measures the level of creatinine in your blood and gives you an estimate of how well your kidneys filter waste. A creatinine urine test can measure creatinine in your urine.

Prothrombine time (PT) is a blood test that measures the time it takes for the liquid portion (plasma) of your blood to clot.

PROCRIT: This medication is used to treat **anemia** (low red blood cell count) in people with long-term serious kidney disease (chronic renal failure), and people receiving chemotherapy for certain types of cancer. It may also be used in anemic patients to reduce the need for blood transfusions before certain planned surgeries that have a high risk of blood loss. Procrit works by signaling the bone marrow to make more red blood cells.

This medication is very similar to the natural substance in your body (erythropoietin) that prevents anemia. This drug was injected on a twice a week basis.

Neupogen This medication is used to increase white blood cell levels in the body. Neupogen is a form of a hormone called granulocyte colony stimulating factor (GCSF). GCSF is a hormone which is produced in the body and is involved in the production of white blood cells.

White blood cells help your immune system work properly. This drug was injected weekly on an as needed basis.

My **MELD SCORE** had been down to 11 from 15 which is quite an improvement, and my viral load was undetectable. According to the Doctors, When your MELD SCORE reaches 25 you are qualified for the transplant procedure.

There are several thousand people waiting on the list, so until you reach a certain level you do not qualify. Some people are so sick by the time they qualify that they do not make it. Then there also has to be a perfect match from a donor.

DONOR OPTIONS: how it works

Sometimes a **living donor** gives up part of their healthy liver to save another's life. This does not happen very often because the risks involved are basically the same to the living donor as to the recipient. Also the living donor must be covered with an insurance policy that will cover them during recovery, or have unlimited funding. So living donors are usually family members who have the same blood type. The Human liver is comprised of two sections.

The right lobe and the left lobe, separated by a ligament (**THE FALCIFORM LIGAMENT**). The Surgeon makes an incision under the rib cage and carefully assess the size of the liver with their own eyes after having seen it with a CT scan. Next, they remove the gallbladder and inject dye into the biliary tree to make sure it is safe for division. Then they dissect the portal vein and artery where it divides the two sides.

They isolate the vein that drains that part of liver and then divide the liver in half very carefully with attention to tying all the blood vessels and bile ducts in that plane. Then the incision it is closed up. The recipient is at this point lying next to the donor and the donor liver is placed into the recipients abdominal cavity. The two patients are sutured back together with dissolvable stitching and staples are placed on the outside of the incision. The liver then re grows to its natural size within a period of weeks.

At this point the donor is recovering from a major abdominal surgery. The first few days will require pain meds. The donor will be given as much pain medication as they need to make them feel comfortable.

The goal is to get them up and out of bed the night of surgery and then walking the hallway the morning after. They can walk down the hallway and see their recipient. They typically receive no blood products and go home about five to six days after surgery.

Approximately one out of three hundred live donors will die, and approximately 30% will have complications.

Deceased (**Cadaver**) Donor Transplant has been a standard way of liver transplantation from the beginning. However, the transplant community has been increasingly suffering from the shortage of donor organs. Patients with advanced liver disease, who do not have the option of a living donor transplant, join the waiting list for a deceased donor.

Unfortunately, over 17,000 to 20,000 Americans on average are currently on the waiting list for a deceased liver transplant with the continuous addition of new patients. In contrast to that high number, the average number of livers that become available for transplantation is around 6,500 a year. Moreover, as a result of the improved safety standards of transportation and violent crimes, the number of organs from previously healthy donors are decreasing and the average age of deceased donors are increasing.

The Human liver is the only major internal body organ that is capable of regeneration. If your liver is not beyond repair and the damage is minimal, you have a good chance of complete recovery. However if there is too much scar tissue or damage you will either die or be transplanted...If you are lucky.

In the not so distant future with the help of these guardian Angels of medicine, vital organs will be manufactured in laboratory cultures. WOW

BETTER ME THAN YOU

December 2012:

On our first visit to Scottsdale, my Wife being a mover and groover in the Las Vegas high end Resort Business wants to have a little fun while we are there. She brings along her Golf Clubs so she can get in a couple of rounds while I am being evaluated.

We stay in the beautiful Golf Community of Fountain Hills. Let me tell you. This gal is top shelf all the way. We had a nice dinner and went back to the Hotel for rest. Being tired and I know she was, we left the clubs and the ice chest in the truck.

I was too weak to lift anything and we had a new TAHOE with all the bells buttons and whistles, so we felt safe locking it up in the parking lot.

Wouldn't you know it. When Vicki went out to the truck the next morning to unload, the golf clubs, ice chest, my cb radio / stereo and my tool bag were gone. They got in to the truck without sounding the alarm, cleaned it out and got away. We were parked just in front of the office. That proves that no matter where you are you are not safe from these people. They had to be extremely talented to pull this off without a hitch. They used our own tools to pull off the heist.....

January 2012:

While being treated with these medications, my Urologist discovered a cyst attached to my testicle on the right side. My scrotum had swollen up and the pain was devastating.

A **Spermatocele**, also known as a spermatic cyst was discovered, They are typically painless, noncancerous (benign) fluid filled cysts that are out pocketing of fluid from the epididymis. They usually sit near the top and/or behind the testicle, but appear separate from the testis. **Spermatoceles** are typically smooth and they are usually filled with a whitish, cloudy fluid and usually contain sperm. Over time, spermatoceles may remain stable in size or they may grow. If in fact the size becomes bothersome or results in pain, then there are several treatment options to rectify the problem. Spermatoceles are generally no more than a nuisance rather than a serious medical condition.

However with the combination of the medicines being taken, and the compromised immune system, the periodic draining caused problems. A decision was made to remove the cyst.

When being treated for HCV they do not suggest any invasive procedures until you are either cured or transplanted. After this operation, which is usually pretty simple and a basic procedure, my health began to deteriorate.

After removal of the cyst, the injectable medications actually started destroying my internal organs. My MELD SCORE started to rise and my **viral load** elevated.

BETTER ME THAN YOU

Your **viral load** is the amount of HCV viruses that you have in a given volume of your blood (usually 1 milliliter = 1 cubic centimeter). More precisely, it means that the amount of Hep C genetic material found in your blood corresponds to as many Hep C viruses as the given number says. Therefore the given number denotes "viral equivalents."

The viral load can range from "non detected" to hundreds of millions. If you are below a certain load amount, you are considered non detected. If your viral level is non-detected you are in fact considered cure. Let me tell you that if you are diagnosed with the **HIDDEN DRAGON,** your life style needs to change immediately. The consumption of alcohol or the carbon monoxide from smoking will kill you quickly. There is no doubt about this. In the following chapters, we will go over some natural and nutritional options that can help you live a healthy and productive life.

However, if cirrhosis has set in you will most likely be candidate for transplant. **EARLY DETECTION AND EVASIVE ACTION IS THE KEY TO SURVIVAL HERE.**

By the time I was transplanted in March 2013, my MELD SCORE was 48. It was the highest in the country.

The estimated 3-month mortality is based on the **MELD** score

40 or more -- 71.3% mortality

30-39 -- 52.6% mortality

20-29 -- 19.6% mortality

10-19 -- 6.0% mortality

<9 -- 1.9% mortality

HCV GENOTYPES: Hepatitis C is divided into six distinct genotypes with multiple subtypes in each genotype class. A genotype is a classification of a virus based on the genetic material in the RNA (Ribonucleic acid) strands of the virus. Generally, patients are only infected with one genotype, but each genotype is actually a mixture of closely-related viruses called quasi-species. These quasi-species have the ability to mutate very quickly and become immune to current treatments, which explains why chronic Hepatitis C is so difficult to treat. The following is a list of the different genotypes of chronic **Hepatitis C**:

Genotype   1a
Genotype   1b
Genotype   2a,   2b,   2c   &   2d
Genotype   3a, 3b, 3c, 3d, 3e & 3f
Genotype 4a, 4b, 4c, 4d, 4e, 4f, 4g, 4h, 4i
&   4j
Genotype   5a
Genotype 6a

Genotype 1 is the most common type of Hepatitis C genotype in the United States and the most difficult to treat. For physicians, knowing the genotype of Hepatitis C is helpful in making a therapeutic recommendation.

Individuals with genotypes 2 and 3 are almost three times more likely than individuals with genotype 1 to respond to therapy with alpha interferon or the combination of alpha interferon and ribavirin. Furthermore, when using combination therapy, the recommended duration of treatment depends on the genotype. For this reason, testing for Hepatitis C genotype is often clinically helpful. Once the genotype is identified, it need not be tested again as genotypes do not change during the course of infection. In my case I was told that my infection was Genotype 2a. I was also informed that my Mother and Father both shared the same chromosomes.

These matching chromosome are apparently a positive chromosome which are apparently the easiest to treat.

THANKS MOM. THANKS DAD.

CHAPTER TWO: OUT OF OPTIONS

It is the day after Christmas December 26th, 2012. I wake up after a night of off and on sleep and spending the day with family / friends. I am groggy and I am trying to put my shoes on. I have absolutely no motor functions and feel like I am being held down by a 1000 lb weight. I can sense the onset of **encephalopathy** coming on. Somehow I manage to make my way to the phone. My dog Chico is crying and can tell that I am in distress. I can't figure out how to get my shoes on. My Wife is at work and my Mother in Law is watching television. Mom is a senior citizen who has suffered a stroke a few years previous, so she is slow at getting around and uses a walker. Dialing 911, I go unconscious. I am admitted to the Hospital in Las Vegas for the 17th time in two years with **hepatic encephalopathy.** My Sister is contacted and rushes to my side in the Hospital.

I am given two transfusions and placed under observation. The hospital staff knows me by my first name and welcomes me once again as a guest. "Howdy Robert" back for another visit huh? This hotel has great service but the prices are extremely high. After three days I stabilize and am sent home. My Wife picks me up and brings me back to the house. I am so happy to see the dogs, and Mom, and proceed to do one of my favorite pastimes. I am watching Football. The play offs are in full swing. And although I don't remember who is playing, I so enjoy watching the excitement. I am daydreaming of when I was strong and healthy. When I could walk and run under my own power and participate in events such as softball, skiing, fishing, camping, working on swimming pools, mowing the lawn, 4 wheeling, working out and so many other of my favorite hobbies and pastimes. I am actually feeling pretty good for a man who is dying.

I am doing my own blood tests, injecting my own antibiotics and keeping my picc line clear.

A PICC line (peripherally inserted central catheter) is a long, thin, flexible tube known as a catheter. It's put into one of the large veins of the arm, near the bend of the elbow. It's then threaded into the vein until the tip sits in a large vein just above the heart.

A **PICC** can be used to give you treatments such as chemotherapy, antibiotics, blood transfusions, intravenous (IV) fluids and liquid nourishment if you're not able to eat. It can also be used to take samples of your blood for testing. This means you won't need to have needles put in every time you have treatment. You can go home with the PICC line in and it can be left in for weeks or months. UNCOMFORTABLE

It is Super Bowl Sunday. February 3, 2013. I wake up suddenly in a pool of blood. I am drowsy and do not know where I am. I am moaning and in pain. I dial 911 on the phone and pass out.

My poor Mother in law is helpless as she listens to the commotion.

When I wake up in the hospital my brother and sister are both there. I am in the emergency room and waiting on a bed. My sister sits next to me as I vomit chunks of blood up in to these bags that are next to my bed. She is comforting me and holding my hand. I am bleeding internally and am given several transfusions while the emergency room staff work relentlessly to save my life. Blood is oozing from all open portals of my body. I am catheterized and put directly in to the intensive care unit. Over the next two weeks I am constantly monitored. The intensive care unit here in Las Vegas has been barely keeping me alive while I fall in and out of coma.

My beautiful niece is there one day when I open my eyes. She is holding my hand and telling me that everything is going to be OK. My adopted nephew who is an accomplished musician comes in and plays me a couple of beautiful classic Led Zeppelin songs on his guitar. The Hospital Clergyman is there several times. I am thinking that my life is over. I believe my family and friends think the same. I have been on the liver transplant list now for over a year and have been back and forth to the Mayo Clinic in Arizona several times. I am ready to die.

The Doctor comes in and tells me there is nothing more they can do for me. I am in dire need of a liver, and Las Vegas does not have the facilities or the technology. Somewhere, someone made a decision to try and transport me to Mayo Clinic. My insurance will not cover the helicopter flight. However it does cover ground transportation.

I am loaded into one of those big ambulances by two of the nicest EMT/ (Paramedics actually) gentleman I have ever met in my life. I am in a state of shock and the pain is unbearable. The EMT who is in the back of the truck with me is administering Morphine constantly to keep me calm and quiet. He is assuring me that I will be OK. When your very survival depends on someone else's skills and training it is a very humbling experience. Phoenix is 300 miles from Las Vegas and it is a four and a half hour drive. These EMT professionals got me there in three hours. I was sliding back and forth in the back of that ambulance like a feather in the wind. I am six foot five and lying in a gurney designed for the average sized human. Quite uncomfortable. They got me there safe.

I was admitted into the Emergency Room at Mayo Clinic Phoenix AZ on February 18th 2013.

I regained consciousness the following morning. I had no Idea where I was.

I could see white entities floating about. Had I died? Are they Angels hovering over me? After my eyes focus, I see that they are Nurses and Doctors.

RELEIF

CHAPTER THREE: THE TRANSPLANT HOUSE

Help In Healing Home (formerly Arizona Transplant House) has been called "a home away from home" by transplant patients and caregivers at Mayo Clinic in Arizona. Since opening the first location at Brusally Ranch in 1999, **Help In Healing Home** has provided housing to more than 4,500 patients and caregivers. Their mission is to provide a caring and healing environment for transplant and cancer patients and their caregivers.

The first 'casita' at The Village at Mayo Clinic was occupied on June 27th, 2009. The second casita was occupied September 8th, 2009 along with the opening of the first Hope Lodge casita. On June 13, 2011, the third casita was occupied bringing the total number of rooms for transplant patients to 18.

Additional casitas will be built as contributions and funding becomes available. Complete Village site plans call for a minimum of 54 guest rooms. So many patients have personally witnessed the hospitality, compassion, and friendliness of the people at Help In Healing Home -- and they regularly request to stay here again upon return visits. If your transplant treatment brings you to Arizona, call them to schedule a tour of The Village at Mayo Clinic in Arizona.

Little could the founders of **Brusally Ranch** have known that their phenomenal house would take on a new life 50 years later. Brusally Ranch was founded shortly after the Tweed family moved to Scottsdale, Arizona in 1949. Named after the combined names of the Tweed's two children, Bruce and Sally, the original ranch located at 84th Street & Cholla in Scottsdale was over 160 acres of land.

This land included a small lake with an island in the middle, the result of a miscalculation on part of the well drillers. It is in this oasis that the Tweeds began to raise and show Arabian horses and became one of the first and most respected families to raise Arabian horses in the United States. And so the Tweed influence continues. Over ten years ago Ed and Ruth's daughter, Sally Groom, donated the Tweed home, the only structure not victim to the bulldozer, to Mayo Clinic Arizona at which time it was transformed into the Arizona Transplant House (now called Help In Healing Home) at Brusally Ranch.

This beautiful facility provided much needed housing and support for the Mayo Clinic's increasing number of organ transplant patients and families.

Help In Healing Home is a special home for special people. Financial contributions help the House provide comfortable and supportive living accommodations. Further assistance comes from memorials, foundation grants, and trusts.

If you are interested in making a financial donation please send your check to:

Help In Healing Home, The Village at Mayo Clinic
5811 E. Mayo Blvd. Phoenix, AZ 85054
Toll Free 1-877-207-3754

You can also donate through their secure online server.
http://www.helpinhealinghome.org/ecomm erce/help-in-healing-home-donation.cfm

They accept Master Card & Visa only.
Donated material goods are always welcomed.
Help In Healing Home is a 501(c)(3) nonprofit organization.

Donations are tax deductible according to the law.

Being in the hospital and not able to make any decisions regarding my health or well being, my family took the reins. My older Brother and his wife had been to the Mayo Clinic with their youngest of two Boys. He had been diagnosed with a rare form of childhood cancer that is known to be quite aggressive. They had stayed at the transplant house while their son was going through treatments and they knew the staff. It was on their recommendation that I was accepted in to the facility. This is a wonderful, beautifully laid out structure of casitas that are laid out in a fashion that enable the patients and their caretakers to be comfortable while waiting on their transplants or going through their cancer treatments. The staff and accommodations are absolutely amazing.

The Village is located on the hospital property, so getting back and forth for treatments is convenient.

Depending on the time of year that you visit the Phoenix / Scottsdale area, long term lodging can be quite expensive. This magical Village is a life saver for those who cannot afford the luxuries of the hotels in the area. Without this facility I would never have been able to afford long term lodging.

CHAPTER FOUR:
IN GOOD HANDS

When I woke up on February 19th I was greeted by a smiling nurse at my bedside. I had just bought a smart phone the week before my last trip in to ICU @ Las Vegas. I had never been a big fan of telephones. The only reason I ever had a cell phone was for work. Up until this point my cell phones were just the basic call in / call out phones. However, with my medical condition being as compromised as it was, I needed the smart phone to keep track of my medical contacts as well as my dosing times for medicine. All of the nurses had the smart phones. So over the next three months while in and out of coma and in and out of the hospital, I received a firsthand crash course on operation of these fascinating communication tools.

The nurses and staff at the Mayo Clinic were there for me whenever I needed anything.

The comparison to the hospitals I had been treated in for over the last two years was like comparing apples to oranges, or the Motel Six to Caesars Palace. The Doctors and Staff at the previous hospitals were trying their best, and they did keep me alive which I appreciate greatly. But the instant feeling of comfort and care, the look on their faces and their positive, professional attitude in Phoenix told me instantly that I was in the right place at the right time.

My kidneys had shut down, as well as my pancreas. I had a picc line put directly in to my jugular vein that threaded its way to just above my heart. This picc line was for blood samples that were being taken two to five times per day, and for administering medications. Another picc line was put in for **kidney dialysis**. **Dialysis** is the artificial process of eliminating waste (diffusion) and unwanted water (ultrafiltration) from the blood. Our kidneys do this naturally.

Some people however, may have failed or damaged kidneys which cannot carry out the function properly. In that event - they may need dialysis. Another reason for the picc lines was that my veins were collapsed from all of the previous blood tests being taken. Scar tissue builds up and makes it almost impossible to insert an IV into the vein.

Along with the multiple medications that I was on, I was also being injected two to four times a day with insulin. After a week of treatment I stabilized and was discharged.

I was feeling fair, although weak and being pushed around in a wheelchair by my Sister and my Wife. I was staying at the Transplant House and going back and forth for my treatments. When my Sister was with me, she was my care taker. When she had to go back to Las Vegas for business my Wife would show up to take charge.

These wonderful gals actually took time off from their jobs and responsibilities to be my personal care givers.

I have no idea what I had done to deserve such dedicated service from them. How do you repay someone who saves your life. **WOW**

Being without the strength to take care of yourself makes you realize just how fragile and how small we are in this Universe. There are so many out there who die before they can be cured. I consider myself the luckiest man on the planet. When I was discharged to the Transplant house I was on quite a few medications. Being weak and unable to administer my own medications, my Sister and my Wife made sure that my meds were taken when needed.

Flowmax 0.4mg orally once per day for the **bladder**

Avodart 0.5mg orally once a day for **testosterone**

Lactulose oral syrup 30ml daily **laxative**

Milk Thistle 500mg orally once per dayfor **liver and kidney function**

1% Vanicream topical ointment apply twice a day for **pruritis**

Rifaximin 550mg orally twice a day for **hepatic encephalopathy**

Freosemide 40mg once per day for **ascites**

Hydroxyzine 25mg four times per day for **pruritis**

Oxycodone 5mg every six hours for **pain**

Pantoprozole 40mg twice a day for **acid reflux**

Zinc Sulfate 220mg twice a day for **immune function**

This is a lot of medicine to be taking. Especially for someone who is not capable of administering it themselves. **Thank God for my Support team.** You cannot miss a dose.

CHAPTER FIVE:
NON TRADITIONAL HELP

There was a time when my Insurance lapsed and I could not afford the luxuries of professional health care. I was retaining water and suffering from **ascites** and **peripheral adema,** as well as **hepatic encephalopathy.** My stomach was also cramping up and I was very tired. I had to find some type of relief. I started talking to a friend at the health food store. The information that I gained there helped me big time while I was waiting on my insurance to kick back in.

1. The first adjustment to make is to **lower your salt / sodium** intake. Our body needs salt to fire the electrolytes that control our brain / heart functions. However, the average American consumes 3000 to 5000 mg of salt per day. Salt makes the body retain water.

When your suffering from ascities and adema salt is a bad thing.
You have to lower your salt intake to maximum 1000mg per day.

2. **Dandelion Root Tea** is helpful in controlling ascites and adema. Dandelion acts as a natural diuretic, causing kidneys to increase the volume of urine and expel the extra salt accumulated inside the body by stimulating more urine production. Dandelion affects the blood volume and water balance in your body, causing excess fluid to move out of the body tissues. The potential changes brought about by the herb in fluid balance, is a reduction in fluid retention and the lowering of the blood pressure. While the exact mechanism of the diuretic effects of dandelion is not well studied, scientists have confirmed that it has strong diuretic activity which is comparable to conventional diuretic drugs. The diuretic effect of dandelion is believed to be due to taraxasterol.

This plant sterol removes fluids from spaces between tissues and the skin.

Dandelion tea tightens the muscles by this action and is often used by bodybuilders for this effect. The herbal extract of dandelion used to make diuretic preparations is taken from the leaves. The roots of the plant are usually used in making herbal laxative. Dandelion is a tonic, a stimulant and a diuretic. It is used to detoxify the kidneys and liver. Topical preparations of the herb are also used to treat skin diseases.

3. **Cut back on animal fats and proteins** to help control **hepatic encephalopathy: Diet:** Doctors advise people to limit how much meat and other animal protein they eat. Toxins (such as ammonia) are formed during the digestion of animal protein, particularly in red meat but also in fish, cheese, and eggs.

To make sure people get enough protein, doctors advise them to eat more foods that contain vegetable protein, such as soy or hemp protein. For Men Whey Protein is suggested.

4. Complex carbohydrates: **complex carbohydrates are made up of at least three single sugar molecules. They include starches, maltose and cellulose.**

Common Complex Carbohydrates

Dairy

- Low fat yogurt

Nuts, Seeds and Legumes

- Lentils
- Kidney beans
- Chick peas
- Split peas
- Soy beans
- Pinto beans
- Rice or Soy Milk

Whole Grain Breads and Pastas

- Breads and pastas made with whole grains provide more fiber.

Consuming Complex Carbohydrates

Consuming carbohydrates is important to ensuring the body has what it needs to operate at peak performance.

These non traditional methods may not be the silver bullet cure. However they can certainly help in the event that you have no other options.

CHAPTER SIX:
THE TRANSPLANT

After being in and out of the hospital several times for tests and procedures, I finally got to the point where I needed 24 hour medical care. I had several, five to be exact **paracentesis** procedures done over the previous year and a half. The pressure build up from ascites caused the formation of two hernias. One was **inguinal**...OUCH. The other was **umbilical**.

Paracentesis: This procedure is performed to drain fluid (ascites) from the abdomen. It is often performed when the fluid build-up becomes uncomfortable for a patient, leading to shortness of breath, reduced appetite, or leg swelling. The procedure involves placing a small catheter (tube) into the abdomen and connecting that tube to a system that drains the fluid into bottles to relieve pressure and for lab testing. This is not a pleasant experience.

Not being able to walk, you are lifted on to a table and the ultrasound technician positions you. Your abdomen is cleaned and dried and an ultrasound is performed. They use a felt tipped marker to mark the target point with an X. A large vinyl patch is placed on your abdomen with a circular hole on the middle. The Doctor then injects a local anesthetic into your abdomen to numb the target area. Then the Doctor inserts a long needle with a surgical hose attached to the end. The needle is carefully inserted, guided by an ultrasound image to the target area.

Care must be taken as to not puncture any internal organs. You must remain absolutely still. If you cough or sneeze you could suffer internal injuries. The fluid is siphoned into glass jars and sent to the lab. At one point of these sessions, they drew 6 liters of fluid out of my abdomen. The next day you are sore at the puncture site. This is not something you want to experience, believe me.

Inguinal hernia: protrudes from the abdomen into the scrotum. An inguinal hernia occurs when soft tissue — usually part of the membrane lining the abdominal cavity (omentum) or part of the intestine — protrudes through a weak point in the abdominal muscles. The resulting bulge can be painful, especially when you cough, bend over or lift a heavy object.

An inguinal hernia isn't necessarily dangerous by itself. It doesn't get better or go away on its own, however, and it can lead to life-threatening complications. Inguinal hernia repair is a common surgical procedure.

Umbilical hernia: occurs when a tissue bulges out through an opening in the muscles on the abdomen near the navel or belly button (umbilicus). About 10% of abdominal hernias are umbilical hernias. For a man in good health these operations are quite simple and non life threatening.

However, when you are on the transplant list and your immune system is compromised they will not operate on you to fix a hernia.

Now you are stuck with the discomfort and pain until after you have healed for a minimum of six months after the liver transplant. This really makes things uncomfortable. As I am fading in and out of coma I see family members and friends at my bedside. I cannot talk. I have a breathing tube in my throat, a catheter in my urethra, an evacuation tube in my anal port, a feeding tube in my nose, a picc line in my right shoulder, a drain tube attached to my abdomen, another picc line in my left chest area for dialysis and an I V drip for hydration. Blood pressure monitor, EKG, and oxygen are also being used.

Once again: IF YOU HAVE HAD A TRANSFUSION PRIOR TO 1993 OR HAVE EVER USED INJECTABLE DRUGS, OR HAVE HAD TATOOS APPLIED BY ANYONE BESIDES A TRAINED PROFESSIONAL IN A STERYL ENVIRONMENT. "GO GET TESTED"

EGD: The procedure: EGD stands for esophagogastroduodenoscopy: right?

This is a test or procedure that is done with a flexible tube with a light and a video camera at the end. This procedure checks for what is known as **Esophageal Varices**. The tube is inserted through the patients mouth. With this test they scan the lining of the esophagus, stomach and first part of small bowel which is known as the duodenum. The patients usually are asleep for this test.

There are always some exceptions. This is not anesthesia but is called "conscious sedation".

There is a slight chance, patients may remember the test or have some discomfort. You are not allowed to eat for twelve hours prior to this procedure.

Esophageal Varices form when blood flow to your liver is obstructed, most often by scar tissue in the liver caused by liver disease. Esophageal varices are abnormal, enlarged veins in the lower part of the esophagus — the tube that connects the throat and stomach. Esophageal varices occur most often in people with serious liver diseases. Esophageal varices develop when normal blood flow to the liver is obstructed by scar tissue in the liver or a clot. Seeking a way around the blockages, blood flows into smaller blood vessels that are not designed to carry large volumes of blood. The vessels may leak blood or even rupture, causing life-threatening bleeding. After this procedure your throat is soar as if you have been coughing for hours on end.

If this condition is not attended to immediately it is quite possible to drown in your own blood.

February 28th, 2013:

My MELD score has elevated to 38, which is among the highest in the country. I am upgraded on the transplant list and my status is critical. Fading in and out of coma and on an intravenous liquid diet I am fading fast. I remember being consoled by clergy on a daily basis. The professional staff, nurses, doctors and techs are the ones in charge of my very existence. I have been told that I am a perfect patient. They have me described as a pleasant 57year old male who's mental status and attitude is exceptional considering his condition. It is mandatory that patients in this condition receive anti depressive medication to relieve stress and the possibility of falling into depression. However the psychiatrist and psychologist have evaluated my condition and diagnosed me as mentally stable.

When I am awake that is. I do not require the anti depressants. My diagnosis is as follows:

1. Blood in Gastric Fundus: **The part of the stomach to the left of the entrance of the esophagus.**

2. End stage liver disease Cirrhosis: A chronic disease of the liver marked by degeneration of cells, inflammation, and fibrous thickening of tissue. It is typically a result of alcoholism or hepatitis.

3. Normocytic anemia: This is iron deficiency anemia ("normo-sit-tic")

4. Hepatic Encephalopathy

5. Ascites and lower extremity Adema

6. Acute kidney failure

7. Hyponatremia: A condition that occurs when the level of sodium in your blood is abnormally low.

8. Pruritus: uncontrollable itching.

9. Thrombocytopenia: the medical term for a low blood platelet count.

10. Benign prostatic Hypotrophy: a common urological condition caused by the non-cancerous enlargement of the prostate gland.

11. Coagulopathy: (also called clotting disorder and bleeding disorder) is a condition in which the blood's ability to clot (coagulate) is impaired.

12. Leucopenia: (also known as leukocytopenia or leucopenia, from Greek λευκός "white" and πενία "deficiency") is a decrease in the number of white blood cells.

Over the next two weeks my condition continues to worsen. I am constantly in and out of COMA. The wait for a liver seems unlikely. I remember watching myself lying in the hospital bed.

It is as if I am viewing myself from the television that is mounted on the wall adjacent to the bed. I can see the whole room from above as the nurses and doctors along with my family and friends enter and exit the ICU room. At this point I am totally unable to get out of bed. The wonderful hospital staff are rotating me and moving me to prevent cramping and bed sores. My gown and bedding is changed twice a day by these dedicated professionals who never give up until the last breath. I can hear them discussing my condition.

The smell and taste of vanilla is pungent to me from the liquid that is being pumped into my body via a nose tube. I have not had solid food of any type in over a week. My skin is as yellow as a banana peel and my blood pressure is 64 / 22. My eyes are inset and as the nurse holds a mirror while she shaves my face.

I remember thinking that I looked like a ZOMBIE. I weigh 145 lbs and I am 6'5". I have lost 100 pounds of muscle mass.

I can see and hear when I am conscious. However talking is impossible. I have been cramped up in a bed that was designed for someone much shorter than myself. Then they find a bed that is designed for a taller person. It feels so comfortable to lie down flat without my knees bent. "Ahhh", there is relief. The smallest addition to my comfort is such a blessing. However, I am not prepared for what is about to happen.

March 10, 2013: There is a liver available. I can remember hearing them talk to my Sister. However they have discovered a staph infection in my blood and they cannot perform the transplant. They need to perform further tests to determine the infection site.

If the infection is in my bloodstream and on its way to the brain, there is a good chance I will not live through this. I am removed from the transplant list for further diagnosis.

Staphylococcus Bacteremia: is an important infection with a very high death rate. Approximately 30% of these patients will die. Comparatively, this accounts for a greater number of deaths than for AIDS, tuberculosis, and viral hepatitis combined. The most consistent predictor of mortality is age, with older patients being twice as likely to die. The impacts of other host factors, including gender, ethnicity, and immune status are unclear. Pathogen-host interactions, especially the presence of shock and the source are strong predictors of outcomes.

Optimal management relies on starting appropriate antibiotics in a timely fashion, resulting in improved outcomes for certain patient subgroups.

The roles of surgery and infectious disease consultations require further study. Although the rate of mortality from this infection is declining, it remains high.

At this point, my **MELD SCORE** is 42. My family from Las Vegas has come. They are there to say their farewells. However, after two days of extensive testing, the results come in. The infection is in one of the **PICC LINES.**

The following diagnosis is directly from the **Infectious Diseases Pathology Report:**

If the patients illness is indeed from a catheter-related Bacteremia, the Ideal solution is to eliminate the PICC catheter and treat with systemic antibiotics. Leaving the catheter in place would require two weeks parenteral therapy as well as lock therapy through the PICC catheter. With respect to reactivating the patient for transplant surgery, the infection must be eliminated ASAP.

Without immediate attention this patient will not survive this dilemma.

A new **PICC LINE** is put in place with a guided x-ray. The guide wire enters through my chest and is threaded to just above the heart.

This is the 4th PICC LINE that has been put into my circulatory system. There are no more target areas available due to collapsed blood veins and low blood pressure. If this doesn't work, its' curtains. The replacement catheter is successful. After three days the infection is eliminated and I am placed back on the available list.

The following report is from medical records 3/16/2013: We discussed with the patients sister the risks, benefits, alternatives, surgery goal, average operation time, length of hospitalization and recovery; risks of surgery including anesthesia, infections, heart attack / stroke possibilities and possible bleed out.

Discussed his long recovery time due to his extremely high MELD SCORE and how ill the patient is at this point.

Discussed his renal function and his need for continued dialysis as well. Wanda understands and wishes to proceed.

THANK YOU SISTER.

At this point I am given 48 hours to live. Somewhere in California, in a State operated Maximum Security Prison facility, there is a 38 year old female who has died. She is in good health and a non violent offender. The warden of the prison contacts the Mayo Clinic and tells them there is a liver available. The blood type is a match. My surgeon sends a flight directly to California with hopes of getting this vital body part back to Phoenix in time. At 8:00 AM on March 17th, 2013 I am wheeled in to the operating room and a complete liver transplant is performed. I can see myself on the table, looking down from above..

The Surgeon and his crew are speaking to each other in soft, monotone medical terms which sound totally familiar to me. I do not know what these medical terms are or what they mean. However, I understand what they are saying. I am not claiming to have experienced an after death experience. However, I am definitely experiencing an out of body experience.

One of several while in the care of these Guardian Angels.

My family and friends are praying for me. I have never been a religious person. I was baptized **Lutheran** as a child. However, my work has occupied my time so that I really never paid much attention to **God**. I guess I figured that I was a pretty good guy and have always been a giver. I have always been more interested in others welfare without much attention to myself. I must have had some good karma coming my way.

The prayers of the people who were concerned for my health must have reached Heaven. It is an absolute miracle that I made it this far. I am forever in debt to the grace bestowed on me while in **God's** hands.

During the transplant procedure the umbilical hernia is repaired and All internal organs are flushed clean with a sterile saline solution.

Six hours and twenty seven minute of **cold ischemia time**. (kold is-KEE-mee-uh ...) In surgery, the time between the chilling of a tissue, organ, or body part after its blood supply has been reduced or cut off and the time it is warmed by having its blood supply restored. This can occur while the organ is still in the body or after it is removed from the body if the organ is to be used for transplantation.

March 18th, 2013:

My eyes open for the first time in 36 hours. I recognize my beautiful Wife immediately. My Sister is next to the bed also. I am conscious and have not talked in over 11 days. I know not where I am or why I am there. After focusing on the environment I recognize my Sister also. She says with a smile on her face " YOU GOT IT BOBBY, YOU GOT IT".

I feel fine and look over at her with a confused look on my face. "YOUR NEW LIVER, IT WAS A SUCCESS".

Tears roll down my face as I realize that I am being tended to by a male nurse who resembles Santa Clause. He is portly and has a bearded face with a smile that lights up the whole room. He is cleaning and re-dressing the drain portal that is protruding from my abdomen. **Now starts the recovery.**

CHAPTER SEVEN RECOVERY:

I look like a cloning experiment from a science fiction movie, or a Cyborg being created in a futuristic setting. HOWEVER, I am stable and breathing under my own power. Seven tubes are hooked up to various parts of my body and the digital, synthesized sounds of medical equipment fill the room. It sounds to me like a symphony of some new form of digital music. I am mentally snapping my fingers and tapping my feet to this music. I flash back to when I was A drummer in a rock band and begin shouting subliminally, "encore, keep playing, percussionist, keep the beat going". When the Nurse comes in for daily maintenance I look down at my body. The staples run from just below my left breast to the right side of my abdomen, just below the rib cage. I have basically been cut in half and put back together.

I hear the doctor tell my Sister that they will be removing the feeding tube from my nose and the breathing tube from my throat soon.

Does this mean I will be able to talk and eat soon? I certainly hope so.

The next procedure is a **Transjugular intrahepatic portosystemic shunt (TIPS),** this is a procedure to create new connections between two blood vessels in your liver. This is not a surgical procedure. It is done by a radiologist using x-ray. A radiologist is a doctor who uses imaging techniques to diagnose and treat diseases.

You will be asked to lie on your back. You will be connected to monitors that will check your heart rate and blood pressure. You will probably receive local anesthesia and medicine to relax you. This will make you pain-free and sleepy. Or, you may have general anesthesia (asleep and pain-free).

Your radiologist will insert a catheter (a flexible tube) through your skin into a vein in your neck.

- On the end of the catheter is a balloon and a metal mesh stent (tube).

- Using x-ray equipment, your radiologist will guide the catheter into a vein in your liver.

- The balloon will be blown up to place the stent. You may feel a little pain when this happens.

- Your radiologist will use the stent to connect your portal vein to one of your hepatic veins.

- At the end of the procedure, your portal vein pressure will be measured to make sure it has gone down.

- After the procedure, a small bandage is placed over the neck area. There are usually no stitches.

- The procedure takes about 60 - 90 minutes to complete.

This new pathway will allow blood to flow better. It will ease pressure on the veins of your stomach, esophagus, intestines, and liver.

Possible risks with this procedure are:

- Damage to blood vessels

- Fever

- Hepatic encephalopathy (a disorder that affects concentration, mental function, and memory, and may lead to coma)
- Infection, bruising, or bleeding
- Reactions to medicines or the contrast dye

- Stiffness, bruising, or soreness in the neck

Rare risks are:

- Bleeding in the belly

- Blockage in the stent

- Cutting of blood vessels in the liver

- Heart problems or abnormal heart rhythms

- Infection of the stent

    After five days of recovery time they are starting to remove hoses and devises. Each time they remove a hose or a sensor there is a huge feeling of relief. I am starting to think that I just might survive this journey after all.

After the first ten days I am whispering and trying to vocalize / talk. My throat is soar from the breathing / feeding tube and my nose is very inflamed from the feeding tube. The physical and recreational therapists are working with me on a daily basis.

The first thing I need to learn is how to sit up. The therapist is there to help train me. After being bed ridden for three months, this is a huge challenge. Once sitting up the next step is standing. I feel as if I will never be able to walk again. However, they are wasting no time pushing me.

I am still catheterized and have not urinated in over eight days. My kidneys are not functioning and dialysis is a painful occurrence three times per week. Being on a liquid diet your body needs to release the water from the blood. Dialysis is the only way to replace kidney function. On day ten there is a urine dribble in to the bag. My kidneys are waking up. However, they are only functioning at 8% so dialysis is continued and the urethral catheter is removed. Standing up to pee is a very exciting goal to set now.   I no longer need the injected insulin because my pancreas has woken up also. My diet consists of broths and sauces.

No solid food and they are conducting **barium swallow tests** on a daily basis. A barium swallow is a test that may be used to determine the cause of painful swallowing, difficulty with swallowing, abdominal pain, bloodstained vomit, or unexplained weight loss.

Barium sulfate is a metallic compound that shows up on X-rays and is used to help see abnormalities in the esophagus and stomach. When taking the test, you drink a preparation containing this solution. The X-rays track its path through your digestive system. After surgery you are not allowed any solid food until you are cleared with a successful swallow test. I am so hungry for a steak right now that it hurts.

You have to be able to get up and move around, use the rest room and shower before they release you from the hospital. With the help of the great, professional, caring staff I am making steady progress.

On March 28th the feeding tube is removed. I am on a diet of sauces, broths and oat meal. The applesauce yogurt and pudding is used to wash down my medications. Water tastes so good and I can feel it hydrating my body with every swallow.

April 5th 2013: I am released from Intensive care and admitted in to the recovery wing of the hospital. The PICC line for medication has been removed and I am eating solid food. I still require Dialysis three days a week, but my kidneys are continuing to improve. In the middle of the Atrium there is a car sitting. It is a Lexus, a new one and the doors are open. I ask the nurse "why is there a car sitting in the hallway?" She tells me that it is used for re-training people to get in and out of a car. I laughed at the thought.

I certainly thought I could get in to a car. I have been driving for over forty years and have always been a good driver.

However, when I tried to get in I could not figure it out. Sure enough, I had to be retrained not only to walk, but to get in and out of a car also. This was a very humbling experience. These therapists and nurses are the absolute best at what they do.

My eyes open to see an Angel. I hear "la la la la ta ta ta ta ra ra ra ra" repeat after me. Next to my bed sits Jennifer Aniston? This nurse I am thinking is an angel. She as a drop dead gorgeous blonde with a smile that eases pain, and the eyes and voice of an Angel. Speech and occupational therapist. I am being trained how to talk, walk and function again. On April 15th I am released and go back to the Transplant House. My visits are on an outpatient basis now and I am feeling better every day.

My Sister and my Wife are still rotating as caretakers and although slow, I can actually get up and down, shower myself, use the bathroom and get dressed on my own now.

April 17th 2013: After lunch I take a fall while navigating to the bathroom. I am 6'5", so when I fall it is TIMBER. I hit the floor pretty hard and bruise my knee. My sister is doing laundry and chatting with some of the tenants.

We have just had lunch and I decided to try to get up on my own. I do not have the strength to get up on my own. When I am helped back to the bed I elevate my leg and doze off. I am awakened with the most intense pain I have ever experienced. My Inguinal hernia has dropped down into my scrotum. I have experienced this before, however this time the pain is unbearable. I am immediately transformed into a helpless child.

The pain from the transplant is nothing compared to this.

A strangulated hernia cuts off blood flow to part of your intestine. This condition is critical, and it can lead to the death of the affected bowel tissue. A strangulated hernia is life-threatening and requires immediate surgery.

After a transplant procedure your doctors will not perform another surgery unless it is a life / death situation. You are at a risk of not surviving anesthesia as well as bleeding out. And on top of that, your body is trying to accept a foreign major internal organ, so all of your healing powers are being concentrated on that one specific area. Once again my wonderful Sister makes a decision to proceed. I am once more unconscious and in critical condition. However, if they do not operate immediately, I will surely die. Immediately after the operation I am put back in the ICU.

After three days I am once again released in to my Sisters care. Man, at this point my body is totally spent. I am back in that friggin wheelchair. Being pushed everywhere I go. The patients and dedication of my Sister and my Wife are unimaginable. As an outpatient, my Sister or my Wife have to drive me to my Dialysis appointments. It is a seven mile drive to the facility, and they conduct themselves so gracefully while caring for me that I am convinced they are both Angels.

Continuing my dialysis three days a week while recovering from multiple operations was a task. Everywhere I go, it is in a wheelchair being pushed by someone else. With absolutely no muscle strength at all you cannot move under your own power. I am now at 130 lbs. At 6 foot 5 that is basically just skin and bones. I need to walk. I need to be able to get around on my own.

After two and a half months of physical therapy and immobility I am back up using a walker. Though weak and fragile, I somehow manage to get back to where I can shower myself and get out of bed using the walker. On June 15th I am released to go home to Las Vegas. I will continue physical therapy and dialysis with hopes that one day I will be strong enough to be independent once more. My Wife has moved us to the other side of town. I am now closer to my doctors as well as my family. This is a gesture that saved me so much time and was so convenient for when my Mother in Law and I were at home alone.

My family could come over almost immediately whenever there was a problem. I would fall and could not get back up. Or Mom would fall and could not get back up. Neither of us were strong enough to help the other back up. It was a fall fest that lasted a couple of months.

Either my family or the paramedics would be at the house on a regular basis helping us back up.

I constantly researched food and nutritional needs to help with the rebuilding of muscle as well as to balance the immune system. It is amazing how much difference it makes when you consume the all natural and organic foods, teas and supplements. Once your body gets used to the quality foods free of pesticides, GMOs and preservatives you will feel a definite improvement of all bodily functions and energy.

Without this change in lifestyle I am certain that I would not be here today.

The in home physical therapist came by twice a week and started me on an exercise program. Before I got sick I could easily lift my own weight 230 lbs plus fifty pounds with no problem. Now I am struggling to lift ten pounds.

However, I had to start somewhere. I was starting to slowly make progress. However, when I was taken to dialysis, I would walk in with a walker and leave in a wheelchair. It was totally exhausting. The dialysis care that I was receiving in Las Vegas was really taking a toll on me. They were pulling too much water out of my blood and dehydrating me.

After being at home for two weeks my health took a turn and it was back to Mayo Clinic. These dedicated life savers had me back up and feeling much better within a few days. Once again I am heading home. I understand why so many die from liver complications. The number one factor is an active support group.

People without families or close friends who jump in and take responsibility for your livelihood are the first to die. It is a full time job being a caregiver for a liver transplant recipient. The second factor is the quality of care.

Not all hospitals or doctors are created equally. The third factor is timing along with a positive attitude and a total understanding of the livers nutritional needs.

After four more months of physical therapy and dialysis, I am strong enough to walk under my own power. Although moving slowly and still weak, I am making good progress. My wife is so busy between her job and taking care of mom that a decision is made for me to make a move. My family owns a nice estate with a Casita in the back garden area. My sister has the Casita completely remodeled and provides me with a safe and secure place to live while recovering. I have bought a car and am driving myself to the store and to medical appointments on a regular basis.

It is a good feeling to be able to get around on my own. In October 2013 I move in to my new home.

My Mother was a local Legend in the Food & Beverage Industry in Las Vegas. My Sister built the Casita for Mom when she retired from the Industry. Mom passed away peacefully in her Casita February 26th, 2008 surrounded by her five children, her grand children and her great grand children. I am truly blessed to have been born in to such a caring and loving family.

I have never thought much about afterlife or paranormal activity. However I know now that there is a connection. Every morning for six months while sleeping my eyes would spring open at 5:00 am and I would be wide awake. I would feel cold chills throughout my body starting at my upper extremities and moving down through my body like an ocean wave. I could smell the perfume Mom used on a daily basis. This would last approximately 30 minutes and then would be gone.

At such time I would fall back asleep and dream of times with Mom. My Mother was 89 years old when she passed away. However, In my dreams she is always in her prime. She is working in the restaurant and still giving me the advice that she so often gave me while working and chatting together. Mom visits me now on a regular basis.

I had told my Sister about a dream where I was receiving a tattoo from a woman. This dream was so real that I remember every little detail. This was also before I knew that my donated liver came from a Woman....IN PRISON. There is definitely a DNA link to all internal organs. It is a memory bank that activates feelings, dreams and traits of the donor. Transferred through the miracle of modern medicine and the unexplainable Human element of miracles.

I am now in recovery two years with no rejection issues or major complications. My organic / natural diet is keeping my bodily functions running at optimum performance. I can no longer do the heavy construction work or long shifts on my feet. However, doing the things I have always dreamed of seem to possibly be within reach. So I do believe that out of all of our falls, when we get back up and put ourselves back on track we can achieve anything.

I am available for consultations or any questions regarding survival or preparation for these issues.

If there is anything I can do to improve the quality of life for any of my brothers and sisters out there I will help in any way possible.

Life after a transplant is a work in progress. It is a job to be taken very seriously. Fifty / 50% of all proceeds from this book go to The Mayo Clinic in Phoenix / Scottsdale Arizona.

My contact info is as follows: I will gladly answer as many emails as humanly possible.,

Dragonbdead13@gmail.com

Robby Robinson

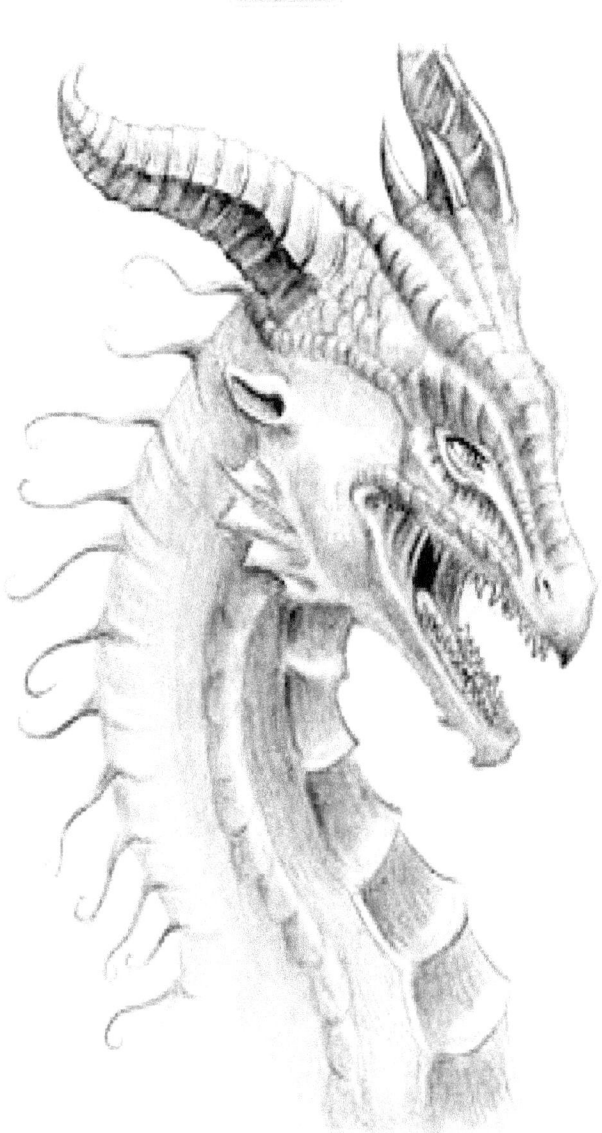

www.ingramcontent.com/pod-product-compliance
Lightning Source LLC
Chambersburg PA
CBHW080643180526

45168CB00008B/3282